THE FERTILITY CRISIS:

How couples can produce offspring without passing through stress.

By

Armstrong smith

TABLE OF CONTENTS

INTRODUCTION

Infertility is a disorder that affects either the male or female reproductive system and is characterized by the inability to obtain pregnancy after twelve months or more of regular sexual activity that is not protected by a protective barrier.

Infertility is a condition that affects millions of people and has repercussions for their families as well as their communities. It is estimated that around one in every six people of reproductive age around the world may experience infertility at some point in their lives.

The most prevalent causes of infertility in the male reproductive system are issues with the ejection of sperm, the absence of sperm or low quantities of sperm, or abnormalities in the shape (morphology) and movement (motility) of the sperm.

The female reproductive system can be affected by a variety of abnormalities, including those that affect the ovaries, uterus, fallopian tubes, and endocrine system, amongst others. Infertility can be caused by these disorders.

It is possible to have primary or secondary infertility. When a person has never been able to conceive a child, they are said to have primary infertility. Secondary infertility, on the other hand, occurs when a person has already conceived at least one child in the past.

Treatment, diagnosis, and prevention of infertility are all things that fall under the umbrella of fertility care. The provision of equal and fair access to fertility care continues to be a challenge in the majority of countries, particularly in countries with low and intermediate incomes. Few national universal health coverage benefit packages give fertility care a higher priority than other medical services.

THE FERTILITY CRISIS

FIRST CHAPTER
WHAT EXACTLY IS THIS INFERTILITY?

One of the medical conditions known as infertility is characterized by the failure of an individual or a couple to obtain a pregnancy or maintain a viable pregnancy after a protracted period of frequent, unprotected sexual intercourse. Infertility can affect both individuals and couples. The condition is often identified after a woman has been trying to conceive for at least a year but has not been successful in doing so on her own. Infertility can be caused by several different variables, some of which include, but are not limited to, physiological problems in one or both spouses, hormone imbalances, structural abnormalities, reproductive system illnesses, or environmental factors. Infertility can be caused by a combination of male and female causes, and it can be caused by difficulties with ovulation, sperm quality and quantity, obstructions in the fallopian tubes, or other reproductive health conditions.

The diagnosis and treatment of infertility are both extremely important tasks that are performed by medical professionals who specialize in reproductive health. Some examples of these doctors include fertility specialists and reproductive endocrinologists. Because of the underlying causes, medical procedures like in vitro fertilization (IVF), fertility drugs, surgery, or changes to one's lifestyle may be needed as possible treatments.

Individuals who are having difficulty conceiving are strongly advised to seek the help of healthcare specialists to receive a specific examination and suitable therapies. It is essential to keep in mind that infertility is a common problem that can be treated.

THE PROBLEM OF INFERTILITY, IS IT?

Infertility stands as a complicated dilemma with far-reaching repercussions that transcend beyond the field of reproductive health. Its influence is enormous, affecting individuals, families, and society at large.

Firstly, on a personal level, infertility can inflict emotional suffering, damage relationships, and undermine one's sense of self-worth and identity. Couples suffering from infertility often experience feelings of despair, anger, and inadequacy as they confront the perceived inability to conceive or bring a pregnancy to term. These mental responsibilities can lead to stress, anxiety, sadness, and even social isolation, worsening the already arduous journey toward parenting.

Moreover, infertility creates considerable financial hardships for affected individuals and families. The costs involved with infertility assessments, treatments, drugs, and assisted reproductive technologies can be excessive, putting a great strain on financial resources. For many, getting specialized fertility treatment remains a privilege rather than a right, compounding socioeconomic inequities in healthcare access and results.

Furthermore, infertility overlaps with broader socioeconomic issues, including cultural norms, gender roles, and reproductive rights. In many countries, there is a pervasive stigma surrounding infertility, spreading myths, misconceptions, and blame. Women, in particular, often face the brunt of societal pressure and criticism surrounding their reproductive capacity, adding to the emotional toll of infertility.

Additionally, the demographic implications of infertility require attention. As birth rates drop in many regions of the world, infertility leads to population aging and demographic imbalances, providing problems for economic growth, healthcare systems, and social welfare programs.

In light of these factors, resolving infertility requires a comprehensive, multidisciplinary strategy that incorporates medical, psychological, social, and ethical components. Initiatives aiming at raising awareness, encouraging education, and lobbying for equal access to fertility care are critical steps towards minimizing the far-reaching impact of infertility on individuals, families, and society. By providing a friendly and inclusive environment, we can create empathy, understanding, and solidarity for those navigating the challenging road of infertility.

CHAPTER TWO
CAUSES OF INFERTILITY

Infertility can result from a multitude of reasons, spanning both physiological and environmental components. Understanding the varied causes of infertility is critical for proper diagnosis and therapy.

Here are some frequent factors contributing to infertility

1. **Ovulation Disorders**: Irregular or missing ovulation might hamper fertility. Conditions such as polycystic ovarian syndrome (PCOS), thyroid abnormalities, and hormonal imbalances can interrupt the ovulation process.

2. **Sperm Disorders**: Issues with sperm production, motility, or morphology can limit fertility in males. Factors include low sperm count, poor sperm quality, genetic abnormalities, and reproductive tract infections that may lead to male infertility.

3. **Fallopian Tube Blockage or Damage**: Blockages or damage to the fallopian tubes can prevent the egg from getting to the uterus for fertilization. This may develop from pelvic inflammatory disease (PID), endometriosis, prior operations, or adhesions.

4. **Uterine or Cervical Abnormalities**: Structural abnormalities within the uterus or cervix can impede implantation or sperm transfer. Conditions such as uterine fibroids, polyps, or cervical stenosis may impact fertility.

5. **Age-related Factors**: Advanced maternal age is associated with a reduced ovarian reserve and decreased egg quality, making conception more difficult. Similarly, growing paternal age can impair sperm quality and raise the likelihood of genetic defects in kids.

6. **Endocrine problems**: Disorders affecting the endocrine system, including diabetes, adrenal problems, and thyroid dysfunction, can disturb hormonal balance and impede fertility.

7. **Lifestyle Factors**: Certain lifestyle decisions can severely affect fertility. These include smoking, excessive alcohol intake, drug use, obesity, poor diet, and exposure to environmental chemicals or pollution.

8. **Genetic Factors**: Genetic abnormalities or chromosomal diseases can contribute to infertility by altering reproductive function or raising the chance of miscarriage.

9. **Unexplained Infertility**: In certain situations, despite rigorous assessment, the cause of infertility remains unexplained. This category, known as unexplained infertility, accounts for a considerable share of infertility cases.

10. **Psychological variables**: Stress, anxiety, and psychological variables can affect fertility by changing hormone levels, menstrual periods, and sexual function.

Understanding the interplay of these factors is critical for personalized fertility screening and treatment techniques, which may include lifestyle modifications, assisted reproductive technologies, fertility drugs, surgical treatments, or counselling assistance. Collaborative efforts between healthcare practitioners and patients are vital in navigating the complex landscape of infertility and optimizing the odds of delivering a healthy pregnancy.

Certainly, infertility risk factors might vary between males and females. Understanding these risk factors is vital for detecting potential difficulties in fertility and treating them effectively. Here are some key risk factors for infertility in both males and females:

Risk Factors for Males

1. **Age**: Advanced paternal age is related to a drop in sperm quality and quantity, which can reduce reproductive potential.

2. **Lifestyle Factors**: Certain lifestyle choices, such as smoking, excessive alcohol consumption, drug usage, and exposure to environmental contaminants, can adversely affect sperm quality and reproductive function.

3. **Medical Conditions**: Chronic illnesses such as diabetes, hypertension, and autoimmune disorders might impair sperm

production and fertility.

4. **Sexually Transmitted Infections** (STIs): Infections such as gonorrhea, chlamydia, and HIV can cause inflammation or scarring of the reproductive organs, leading to infertility.

5. **Genetic Factors**: Genetic disorders such as Klinefelter syndrome, Y chromosome deletions, and chromosomal aberrations might impact sperm production and fertility.

6. **Varicocele**: A varicocele is a swelling of the veins that drain the testicle and is a common cause of diminished sperm production and quality.

7. **Testicular Trauma or Surgery**: Injuries to the testicles or surgical procedures in the genital area might affect sperm production or disturb reproductive function.

8. **Obesity:** Excess body weight and obesity have been linked to hormonal imbalances and poor sperm quality.

Risk Factors for Females

1. **Age**: Advanced maternal age is associated with deteriorating ovarian reserve and decreased egg quality, leading to diminished fertility and an increased risk of miscarriage.

2. **Ovulatory abnormalities**: Conditions such as polycystic ovary syndrome (PCOS), thyroid abnormalities, and hormonal imbalances can interrupt ovulation and affect fertility.

3. **Endometriosis**: Endometriosis, a disorder where tissue comparable to the lining of the uterus grows outside the uterus, can cause pelvic pain and infertility by damaging the ovaries, fallopian tubes, and uterus.

4. **Pelvic Inflammatory Disease** (PID): PID, commonly caused by sexually transmitted infections such as chlamydia or gonorrhea, can lead to scarring and damage to the reproductive organs, resulting in infertility.

5. **Uterine or Cervical Abnormalities**: Structural abnormalities in the uterus or cervix, such as uterine fibroids, polyps, or cervical stenosis, can impede implantation or sperm transfer.

6. **Blocked Fallopian Tubes**: Blockages or damage to the fallopian tubes can prevent the egg from meeting the sperm, resulting in

infertility.

7. **Previous Surgeries**: Surgeries involving the reproductive organs, such as ovarian cystectomy or tubal ligation reversal, might increase the risk of scarring and adhesions, compromising fertility.

8. **Lifestyle variables**: Similar to males, lifestyle variables including smoking, excessive alcohol use, drug usage, obesity, and exposure to environmental contaminants can significantly affect female fertility.

Identifying and managing these risk factors through lifestyle modifications, medical interventions, and reproductive treatments can enhance fertility results for people and couples encountering issues with conception.

How infertility can be tested by both males and females

Certainly! Testing for infertility often entails a battery of diagnostic evaluations to discover potential variables contributing to difficulties in conception. Here's an overview of common testing for both males and females.

Testing for males

1. **Semen Analysis:** This is the major test to evaluate male fertility. It entails testing a semen sample for factors such as sperm count, motility (movement), morphology (shape), and volume. Abnormalities in these measures may suggest underlying reproductive difficulties.

2. **Hormone Testing:** Blood tests can examine hormone levels, including testosterone, follicle-stimulating hormone (FSH), luteinizing hormone (LH), and prolactin. Hormonal abnormalities can impair sperm production and reproductive function.

3. **Genetic Testing:** Genetic tests may be undertaken to screen for chromosomal abnormalities, Y chromosome deletions, or genetic mutations that could impair fertility.

4. **Physical Examination:** A physical examination of the

genitals and reproductive organs may help discover structural abnormalities, varicoceles (swollen veins in the scrotum), or other diseases that could compromise fertility.

5. **Specialized Testing:** In some circumstances, additional testing such as scrotal ultrasonography, sperm DNA fragmentation analysis, or testicular biopsy may be recommended to further assess reproductive difficulties.

Testing for females:

1. **Ovulation Assessment**: Monitoring menstrual cycles, basal body temperature charting, and ovulation predictor kits can assist in identifying if ovulation is occurring regularly.

2. **Hormone Testing:** Blood tests can check hormone levels, including follicle-stimulating hormone (FSH), luteinizing hormone (LH), estradiol, progesterone, and thyroid hormones, to determine ovarian function and hormonal balance.

3. **Pelvic Ultrasound:** Transvaginal ultrasound imaging can help check the shape of the uterus, ovaries, and fallopian tubes and detect any abnormalities such as fibroids, ovarian cysts, or polyps.

4. **Hysterosalpingography** (HSG): This method involves injecting a contrast dye into the uterus and fallopian tubes while doing X-ray imaging. It helps examine the morphology of the uterus and discover blockages or anomalies in the fallopian tubes.

5. **Laparoscopy**: In cases where endometriosis or pelvic adhesions are suspected, a laparoscopic procedure may be performed to directly visualize and analyze the pelvic organs.

6. **Ovarian Reserve Testing**: Blood tests such as anti-Müllerian hormone (AMH) and antral follicle count (AFC) can provide insights into a woman's ovarian reserve and potential for pregnancy.

7. **Genetic Testing:** Genetic screening may be suggested to identify chromosomal abnormalities or genetic mutations that could influence fertility or raise the risk of certain reproductive problems.

By undergoing these diagnostic procedures, healthcare experts can discover underlying causes contributing to infertility and establish personalized treatment regimens tailored to the specific needs of individuals and couples. Early and precise diagnosis is crucial to maximizing reproductive outcomes and achieving a successful pregnancy.

Certainly! Solutions for infertility depend on the underlying problems found during diagnostic tests. Treatment approaches try to treat specific concerns and optimize the chances of conception. Here are extensive answers for infertility in both males and females:

Solutions for males:
1. Lifestyle Modifications
Encourage healthier lifestyle choices such as stopping smoking, limiting alcohol use, keeping a healthy weight, and minimizing exposure to environmental contaminants.

2. Medications
Hormonal therapies: In cases of hormonal imbalances, hormone replacement therapy or drugs such as clomiphene citrate may be administered to boost sperm production.
Antibiotics: If an infection is found, antibiotics can help address the underlying cause.

3. Surgical interventions
Varicocele repair: Surgical correction of varicoceles, which are bulging veins in the scrotum, may enhance sperm production and quality.
When there are no sperm in the ejaculate because of a blockage, this is called obstructive azoospermia. To get sperm for assisted reproductive techniques, surgery like testicular sperm extraction (TESE) or microsurgical epididymal sperm aspiration (MESA) may be needed.

4. Assisted Reproductive Technologies (ART).
Intrauterine insemination (IUI): Sperm are cleaned and concentrated before being inserted directly into the woman's uterus during ovulation.

In vitro fertilization (IVF) and intracytoplasmic sperm injection (ICSI): IVF involves fertilizing eggs with sperm in a laboratory setting, while ICSI involves injecting a single sperm directly into an egg. Both procedures can bypass specific male infertility causes and facilitate conception.

5. Genetic Counselling:

Couples with genetic abnormalities or inherited illnesses may benefit from genetic counselling to understand the risks to offspring and investigate solutions such as preimplantation genetic testing (PGT) during I Solutions for Females.

1. Lifestyle Modifications:

Emphasize healthy lifestyle behaviors, including keeping a balanced diet, frequent exercise, managing stress, and avoiding tobacco, alcohol, and illicit drugs.

2. Medications:

Ovulation induction: Fertility drugs such as clomiphene citrate, letrozole, or gonadotropins may be recommended to stimulate ovulation in women with ovulatory problems.

Hormonal therapies: Hormonal treatments may be used to control menstrual cycles and repair hormonal imbalances.

3. Surgical interventions:

Laparoscopic surgery: Surgical procedures may be performed to treat diseases such as endometriosis, ovarian cysts, fibroids, or pelvic adhesions that might impede fertility.

Hysteroscopic surgery: Minimally invasive techniques can address uterine anomalies such as polyps, fibroids, or septum, which may interfere with implantation or conception.

4. Assisted Reproductive Technologies (ART):

Intrauterine insemination (IUI): IUI may be indicated as a first-line treatment for women with unexplained infertility or cervical issues.

In vitro fertilization (IVF) and related techniques: IVF and related techniques like intracytoplasmic sperm injection (ICSI) and preimplantation genetic testing (PGT) can help women who are having trouble getting pregnant get past a number of problems.

5. Egg Donation or Surrogacy:

For women with decreased ovarian reserve or other reproductive issues, obtaining donated eggs or considering surrogacy may be possibilities for achieving conception.

6. Counselling and Support:

Emotional support and counselling programs can help individuals and couples cope with the emotional stress and problems involved with infertility treatment.

By addressing the specific reasons contributing to infertility and adapting treatment approaches to individual needs, healthcare providers can enhance reproductive results and support individuals and couples on their journey to motherhood. Collaboration between patients, healthcare professionals, and fertility specialists is crucial to navigating the intricacies of infertility therapy and ensuring a successful pregnancy.

CHAPTER THREE

IS INFERTILITY CURABLE?

Infertility is a complex medical issue, and whether it is curable depends on several aspects, including the underlying reasons, the individual's health status, and accessible treatment choices. Here's a nuanced perspective:

Yes, infertility can be curable.

1. **Causes that can be found:** If an infertility problem is caused by something that can be treated, like an imbalance of hormones, an infection, or a problem with the structure of the body, specific medical treatments, lifestyle changes, or surgery may be able to fix the problem and restore fertility.

2. **Changes in Reproductive Medicine:** New technologies in assisted reproductive technologies (ART) like in vitro fertilization (IVF), intracytoplasmic sperm injection (ICSI), and preimplantation genetic testing (PGT) have completely changed the way fertility care is provided. These treatments offer feasible solutions for people and couples facing diverse infertility issues, considerably enhancing the odds of conception and pregnancy.

3. **Multidisciplinary Approach:** Comprehensive fertility evaluation and treatment often entail a multidisciplinary approach that blends medical knowledge, counselling assistance, and lifestyle changes. By addressing the physical, emotional, and psychological components of infertility, healthcare providers can enhance treatment outcomes and accompany patients throughout their fertility journey.

No, Infertility May Not Be Curable:

1. **Unidentified or unmodifiable variables:** In some situations, infertility may develop from variables that are difficult to identify or alter, such as severe age-related loss in ovarian reserve, genetic predispositions, or irreparable injury to reproductive organs.

While therapies like IVF can help overcome certain impediments to conception, they may not always result in a successful pregnancy, particularly in situations of severe infertility.

2. **Personal Variability:** Fertility outcomes can vary greatly across individuals and couples, depending on factors such as age, overall health, genetic predispositions, and response to therapy. Despite rigorous diagnostic and treatment efforts, some individuals may not achieve a successful conception or may require numerous treatment cycles before obtaining a pregnancy.

3. **Emotional and Financial Considerations:** Coping with infertility can be emotionally and financially hard, particularly when treatment options are limited or unsuccessful. The emotional toll of infertility, coupled with the financial weight of fertility treatments, can compound stress and anxiety for people and couples navigating the reproductive path.

In conclusion, while infertility may be cured or controlled for some individuals through focused therapies and breakthroughs in reproductive health, it remains a complicated and diverse disease with no one-size-fits-all answer. Each case of infertility is unique, needing specialized evaluation, treatment planning, and continuous support to enhance reproductive outcomes and satisfy the various requirements of patients.

How can traditional therapies support curing infertility?

Traditional therapies, frequently anchored in cultural customs and herbal therapy, have been applied for ages to manage numerous health concerns, including infertility. While the success of traditional treatments in resolving infertility may vary, some proponents offer many ways in which these remedies might help:

1. **Hormonal Balance:**
Certain herbs and natural therapies are considered to support hormonal balance, which is necessary for regular ovulation in women and optimal sperm production in men. Herbs like chasteberry (Vitex agnus-castus) and maca root (Lepidium

meyenii) are widely used to regulate menstrual cycles and enhance reproductive health.

2. Nutritional Support:

Traditional therapies frequently emphasize the use of nutrient-rich herbs and foods to improve overall health and fertility. Ingredients such as royal jelly, bee pollen, ginseng, and ginkgo biloba are considered to boost vitality and reproductive function.

3. Stress Reduction:

Many traditional therapies combine relaxation techniques, meditation, and herbal cures recognized for their calming effects. Stress reduction is vital for fertility, as high levels of stress hormones can interfere with reproductive hormones.

4. Improved blood circulation:

Traditional treatments like acupuncture and traditional Chinese medicine (TCM) highlight the necessity of ensuring healthy blood circulation to the reproductive organs. Acupuncture, in particular, is believed to promote blood flow to the uterus and ovaries, potentially enhancing ovarian function and uterine lining thickness.

5. Detoxification:

Some traditional therapies involve herbal formulations and dietary regimens targeted at detoxifying the body and removing toxins that may interfere with reproductive function. Detoxification is considered to enhance general health and optimize fertility.

6. Libido Enhancement:

Certain herbs and therapies are considered to stimulate libido and sexual performance, which can raise the odds of conception. Aphrodisiac herbs, including ginseng, maca root, and Tribulus terrestris, are widely used for this purpose.

7. Supporting Traditional Beliefs and Practices:

For many individuals and societies, traditional treatments carry important cultural and spiritual relevance. The belief in the efficacy of these therapies might provide emotional and psychological support, which may indirectly improve reproductive outcomes.

It's crucial to emphasize that while traditional remedies may offer potential benefits, they should not be considered a substitute for evidence-based medical therapies. It's suggested for individuals and couples experiencing infertility to contact certified healthcare practitioners and fertility specialists for full evaluation, diagnosis, and treatment choices customized to their personal needs. Integrating traditional remedies with current medical treatments under the guidance of healthcare professionals may offer a holistic approach to reproductive care. Additionally, it's necessary to be vigilant about potential side effects and combinations with conventional medications when using traditional therapies.

Treatment for infertility in both males and females

The infertility treatment differs based on the underlying factors found through diagnostic tests. Here's an overview of therapy possibilities for both males and females:

Treatment for Males:

1. Lifestyle Modifications:

Encourage healthier lifestyle choices, including quitting smoking, limiting alcohol intake, keeping a healthy weight, and minimizing exposure to environmental pollutants.

2. Medications:

Hormone therapy: If hormonal imbalances are found, medicines such as clomiphene citrate or gonadotropins may be recommended to enhance sperm production.

3. Surgery:

Varicocele repair: Surgical correction of varicoceles may improve sperm quality and quantity.

In cases of obstructive azoospermia, surgical methods such as testicular sperm extraction (TESE) or microsurgical epididymal sperm aspiration (MESA) can be used to get sperm for assisted reproductive technologies.

4. Assisted Reproductive Technologies (ART):

Intrauterine insemination (IUI): Concentrated sperm is directly injected into the woman's uterus during ovulation.

In vitro fertilization (IVF) and intracytoplasmic sperm injection (ICSI): IVF involves fertilizing eggs with sperm in a laboratory, while ICSI involves injecting a single sperm directly into an egg. Both procedures can overcome numerous male fertility concerns.

5. Genetic Counselling:

Couples with genetic abnormalities may benefit from genetic counselling to determine the risk of passing on genetic disorders to their offspring.

Treatment for females:

1. Lifestyle Modifications:

Emphasize good lifestyle practices, including keeping a balanced diet, regular exercise, managing stress, and avoiding tobacco, alcohol, and illicit drugs.

2. Medications:

Ovulation induction: Fertility medicines such as clomiphene citrate, letrozole, or gonadotropins may stimulate ovulation.

Hormone therapy: Medications may be recommended to control menstrual cycles and treat hormonal imbalances.

3. Surgery:

Laparoscopic surgery: Surgical techniques may cure diseases such as endometriosis, ovarian cysts, fibroids, or pelvic adhesions.

Hysteroscopic surgery: Minimally invasive techniques can address uterine anomalies such as polyps, fibroids, or a septum.

4. Assisted Reproductive Technologies (ART):

Intrauterine insemination (IUI): IUI may be indicated as a first-line treatment for unexplained infertility or cervical causes.

In vitro fertilization (IVF) and related techniques (IVF, ICSI, and preimplantation genetic testing (PGT)) can solve numerous female fertility difficulties.

5. Egg Donation or Surrogacy:

For women with decreased ovarian reserve or other problems, using donated eggs or considering surrogacy may be a possibility to achieve conception.

6. Counselling and Support:

Emotional support and counselling programs can help individuals and couples cope with the emotional stress and problems involved with infertility treatment.

Treatment plans are generally personalized, taking into account the specific circumstances contributing to infertility. Collaboration between patients, healthcare providers, and fertility specialists is vital to navigating the complexity of infertility treatment and optimizing the odds of a successful conception. Regular follow-up meetings and open communication help change treatment strategies based on individual reactions and circumstances.

Types of exercise to help prevent infertility

Exercise is a crucial component of a healthy lifestyle that can contribute to enhancing fertility in both men and women. Here are some types of exercise that can help alleviate infertility:

For Men:

1. Aerobic Exercise:

Activities such as jogging, brisk walking, cycling, and swimming can improve cardiovascular health and promote blood flow throughout the body, including the reproductive organs. Improved blood circulation to the testes can support healthy sperm production and quality.

2. Strength Training:

Resistance exercises like weightlifting, bodyweight exercises, and resistance band workouts help improve muscle strength and support hormonal balance. Strength training boosts testosterone production, which is required for sperm formation and reproductive function.

3. Yoga and stretching:

Yoga and stretching exercises can help reduce tension, increase flexibility, and promote relaxation. Certain yoga poses, such as the Cobra Pose (Bhujangasana) and the Butterfly Pose (Baddha

Konasana), target the pelvic area and encourage blood flow to the reproductive organs.

For Women:

1. **Low-Impact Cardiovascular Exercise:**

Low-impact exercises such as walking, swimming, cycling, and using elliptical machines are soft on the joints and can enhance cardiovascular health. Regular cardiovascular activity stimulates blood circulation, supports hormonal balance, and enhances ovulation.

2. **Yoga and Pilates:**

Yoga and Pilates focus on strengthening the core muscles, improving flexibility, and fostering relaxation. Certain yoga poses, such as the Bridge Pose (Setu Bandhasana) and the Reclining Bound Angle Pose (Supta Baddha Konasana), might help enhance blood flow to the pelvic region and boost reproductive health.

3. **Mind-Body Exercises:**

Mind-body exercises such as tai chi, qigong, and meditation help lower stress, anxiety, and cortisol levels, which can positively improve fertility. Mindfulness activities increase emotional well-being and create a suitable environment for conception.

4. **Pelvic Floor Exercises:**

Pelvic floor exercises, commonly known as Kegel exercises, assist in strengthening the muscles of the pelvic floor. Strong pelvic floor muscles assist the reproductive organs, improve bladder control, and promote sexual performance.

5. **Dance and Aerobic Workouts:**

Dance-based workouts and aerobic exercises like Zumba, dance cardio, and aerobics courses give a fun and effective approach to improving cardiovascular health, burning calories, and maintaining a healthy weight, which is vital for fertility.

It's crucial to find exercises that you enjoy and that meet your fitness level and interests. Aim for a balanced fitness regimen that incorporates cardiovascular workouts, weight training, flexibility exercises, and stress-reducing activities. Consulting with a healthcare specialist or fitness professional before starting a new exercise program is encouraged, especially for people with unique health concerns or fertility issues. Remember that consistency and moderation are crucial to attaining optimal health and reproductive benefits from exercise.

Exercise can play a key role in boosting fertility and enhancing reproductive health in both men and women. Here's how exercising helps decrease infertility:

For Men:

1. Improves Sperm Quality:

Regular physical exercise has been associated with increased sperm quality, including a higher sperm count, motility, and morphology. Exercise helps optimize testosterone levels and reduce oxidative stress, which can significantly improve sperm production and function.

2. Reduces stress and anxiety:

Exercise is a natural stress reliever and mood enhancer. High levels of stress and anxiety can significantly influence sperm production and hormonal balance. Engaging in regular exercise helps lower stress hormones and enhances general mental well-being, which can boost fertility outcomes.

3. Promotes healthy weight management:

Obesity and excess body weight are connected with hormonal abnormalities and impaired fertility in males. Exercise helps maintain a healthy weight and minimizes the risk of obesity-related diseases such as insulin resistance and metabolic syndrome, which can affect reproductive function.

4. Enhances Blood Circulation:

Regular exercise promotes blood circulation throughout the body, including the reproductive organs. Enhanced blood flow to the testes enhances nutrient delivery and oxygenation, promoting optimal sperm generation and function.

For Women:

1. Regulates menstrual cycles:

Exercise helps regulate menstrual periods by promoting hormonal balance and boosting ovulation. Women who engage in regular physical exercise are less likely to develop irregular periods or ovulatory problems, which can contribute to infertility.

2. **Reduces the risk of Polycystic Ovary Syndrome** (PCOS):

PCOS is a prevalent cause of female infertility characterized by hormonal abnormalities, irregular periods, and ovarian cysts. Exercise plays a critical role in preventing and controlling PCOS by improving insulin sensitivity, lowering androgen levels, and boosting ovulation.

3. **Supports healthy weight management:**

Maintaining a healthy weight is vital for fertility in women. Obesity and excess body fat can disturb hormonal balance, interfere with ovulation, and raise the risk of infertility. Regular exercise, together with a balanced diet, helps manage weight and optimize reproductive function.

4. **Enhances Psychological Well-Being:**

Infertility can have a toll on mental health and emotional well-being. Exercise is a natural mood enhancer and stress reducer, helping women cope with the emotional obstacles of infertility treatment and boosting general psychological resilience.

5. **Improves Blood Circulation to Reproductive Organs:**

Physical exercise promotes blood flow to the uterus and ovaries, which supports follicle development, implantation, and general reproductive health.

It's crucial to note that, while exercise might be beneficial for fertility, moderation is key. Excessive or vigorous exercise, especially in women, might have the opposite effect and disrupt menstrual cycles or ovulation. Consulting with a healthcare professional or reproductive specialist before starting an exercise plan is recommended, especially for people with unique health concerns or fertility issues. Additionally, combining exercise with other lifestyle improvements such as a balanced diet, enough sleep, and stress management skills can further help reproductive goals.

How infertility causes mental issues in our civilizations
Infertility can have a dramatic influence on mental health, often leading to a range of emotional struggles and psychological discomfort for individuals and couples facing difficulties conceiving.

CHAPTER FOUR

HOW INFERTILITY MIGHT CAUSE MENTAL HEALTH PROBLEMS

1. Emotional distress:
Coping with infertility can provoke a range of deep feelings, including sadness, grief, frustration, rage, and disappointment. The failure to conceive or maintain a pregnancy can test one's sense of self-worth and identity, leading to feelings of inadequacy and despair.

2. Stress and anxiety:
The uncertainty and unpredictability of the fertility quest can be tremendously stressful. Fertility therapies, medical procedures, and the financial burden of infertility can worsen stress and anxiety levels. Each cycle of treatment offers optimism, anticipation, and the fear of potential letdown.

3. Depression:
Chronic stress and unresolved loss linked to infertility might contribute to depression. Feelings of sadness, hopelessness, and despair may intensify with time, hurting the overall mood and quality of life.

4. Social Isolation and Stigma:
Infertility can lead to feelings of isolation and social disengagement, particularly when friends, family, or society at large do not understand or respect the emotional intricacies of infertility. The prevalent stigma surrounding infertility may further compound feelings of guilt and loneliness.

5. Relationship Strain:
Infertility can strain relationships, leading to disagreements, communication breakdowns, and emotional distance between couples. Differences in coping styles, expectations, and fertility

treatment options can create friction and strain the partnership.

6. Negative Self-Image:

Infertility can significantly affect self-esteem and body image, particularly for women whose femininity and sense of womanhood may be tightly related to their capacity to conceive and bear children. Men may also experience sentiments of emasculation and inadequacy.

7. Coping Mechanisms:

Individuals and couples struggling with infertility may resort to unhealthy coping techniques such as substance misuse, overeating, or isolation from social activities, which can further exacerbate mental health problems.

8. Unresolved Grief and Loss:

Infertility can be accompanied by feelings of sadness and loss, particularly for individuals who encounter failed fertility treatments, pregnancy losses, or the inability to produce biological children. Unresolved grief can impair mental health and emotional well-being.

9. Impact on Future Plans and Goals:

Infertility can interrupt life plans and goals, prompting individuals and couples to reassess their aspirations, hopes, and expectations for the future. Uncertainty about motherhood and family-building can produce existential sorrow and distress.

It's crucial to realize the emotional toll of infertility and seek support from healthcare specialists, mental health professionals, support groups, and loved ones. Counselling, therapy, and support programs can assist people and couples in negotiating the emotional obstacles of infertility, creating skills, and fostering resilience in the face of hardship. By addressing the psychological aspects of infertility, individuals and couples can strive towards healing, acceptance, and a sense of empowerment on their reproductive journey.

A general comment on infertility in our societies

Contributions to infertility involve diverse activities intended to raise awareness, lobby for access to care, improve research, and provide support to individuals and couples afflicted by infertility.

Here are numerous contributions in the domain of infertility:

1. Awareness Campaigns:

organizing and participating in awareness initiatives to educate the public about the prevalence, causes, and impact of infertility. These advertisements help minimize stigma, boost understanding, and foster empathy towards individuals and couples with fertility issues.

2. Advocacy for Access to Care:

advocating for increased access to fertility testing, treatments, and support services. This involves pushing for insurance coverage for infertility treatments, decreasing financial barriers, and fighting for policies that support reproductive health and family-building alternatives.

3. Support Groups and Resources:

Establishing and facilitating support groups, internet forums, and community resources for people and couples battling infertility. These networks offer emotional support, information sharing, and a sense of community among people navigating the fertility path.

4. Fertility Education and Counselling:

providing comprehensive fertility education, counselling, and preconception care to individuals and couples. Fertility education programs empower individuals to make informed decisions about their reproductive health, grasp fertility preservation alternatives, and optimize their chances of conception.

5. Research and Innovation:

Supporting research programs focus on expanding our understanding of infertility causes, treatments, and outcomes. Funding research studies, clinical trials, and novel technology accelerates development in reproductive science and increases treatment options for individuals and couples.

6. Fertility Preservation:

Promoting knowledge and access to fertility preservation options for those experiencing medical treatments or diseases that may compromise fertility. Fertility preservation treatments such as egg freezing, sperm banking, and embryo cryopreservation give promise for future family-building choices.

7. Cultural and Societal Change:

challenging cultural norms, societal expectations, and misconceptions around infertility. Advocating for inclusive language, destigmatizing infertility, and promoting diverse family-building paths contribute to a more supportive and understanding culture.

8. Holistic Support Services:

providing holistic support services that address the physical, emotional, and psychological aspects of infertility. Integrative care models that combine medical treatments with alternative therapies, counselling, nutrition assistance, and stress management strategies can boost general well-being and fertility outcomes.

9. Fertility Preservation for Cancer Patients:

supporting projects that give fertility preservation options for cancer patients before undertaking therapies that may compromise fertility. Fertility preservation counselling and services give hope for parenthood after cancer therapy.

10. Legislative and Policy Advocacy:

advocating for legislation and regulations that safeguard reproductive rights, ensure access to fertility treatments, and ban discrimination based on reproductive status. Legislative lobbying initiatives help shape healthcare legislation and promote reproductive justice for all people and couples.

These efforts collectively attempt to address the complex difficulties of infertility, promote equity in access to care, and develop supportive communities that empower individuals and couples on their fertility journey.

CHAPTER FIVE

HOW INFERTILITY HAS AFFECTED THE GLOBAL IMPACT

Infertility has far-reaching ramifications on a worldwide scale, affecting individuals, families, communities, and societies in a variety of ways, including the following:

1. **Population Dynamics:** Infertility can affect population dynamics by affecting fertility rates and population growth. There is a possibility of demographic shifts occurring in areas where the rates of infertility are high and where access to fertility therapy is restricted. These shifts may include populations that are getting older and birth rates that are decreasing.

2. **Healthcare Systems:** Infertility creates enormous demands on healthcare systems, necessitating the allocation of resources for diagnostic tests, fertility therapies, and support services. In countries where infertility treatments are not covered by insurance or where access to specialized care is limited, patients may confront financial barriers to treatment.

3. **Economic Impact:** Infertility can have economic effects at both the individual and social levels. Fertility treatments and assisted reproductive technologies (ART) can be costly, inflicting financial hardship on people and families. Lost productivity owing to time off work for reproductive treatments and associated stress can also harm economic production.

4. **Psychological and Emotional Well-being:** Infertility can have profound psychological and emotional repercussions on people and couples. The emotional toll of infertility, including stress, worry, despair, and bereavement, can influence mental health and general well-being. Addressing the psychological components of infertility is vital for complete patient care.

5. **Social Stigma and Cultural Norms:** Infertility may be

stigmatized in particular cultures and societies, leading to social isolation, humiliation, and prejudice. Societal expectations surrounding children and traditional gender roles can increase the stigma associated with infertility, placing additional emotional pressures on individuals and couples.

6. **Reproductive Rights and Access to Care:** Infertility presents crucial problems linked to reproductive rights and access to care. In many parts of the world, access to fertility treatments, reproductive health services, and family planning tools is limited, particularly for vulnerable groups. Advocacy activities are essential to providing fair access to fertility care for all individuals and couples.

7. **Global Health and Development:** Infertility connects with broader global health and development goals, including initiatives to improve maternal and child health, reduce infant mortality, and promote gender equality. Addressing infertility as a public health issue involves comprehensive solutions that promote access to affordable, quality healthcare services and reproductive rights.

8. **Research and Innovation:** Infertility research and innovation fuel improvements in reproductive medicine, genetics, and assisted reproductive technologies. Collaborative efforts among researchers, healthcare providers, politicians, and advocacy organizations are vital for expanding scientific understanding, enhancing treatment outcomes, and resolving global infertility concerns. In summary, infertility has numerous ramifications that extend beyond individual experiences to impact healthcare systems, economics, social norms, and global health goals. Addressing the complex issues of infertility requires a coordinated, multidisciplinary strategy that incorporates medical, social, cultural, and ethical factors to promote equitable access to care and support reproductive rights for all persons and couples.

CONCLUSIONS ON INFERTILITY

Infertility is a multidimensional issue that can have profound physical, emotional, and social repercussions for individuals and couples worldwide. Concluding comments on infertility frequently reflect the intricacies and nuances inherent in navigating the fertility path.

Here are numerous major conclusions:

1. **Infertility is a Common and Diverse Challenge:**
Infertility affects millions of individuals and couples globally, irrespective of age, race, ethnicity, or financial condition. Its causes are numerous and multifaceted, spanning medical, genetic, environmental, and lifestyle variables.

2. **The emotional toll of infertility is significant.**
Coping with infertility can generate a range of deep feelings, including sadness, grief, frustration, worry, and despair. The emotional toll of infertility extends beyond the person to influence relationships, self-esteem, and overall well-being.

3. **Access to care and support is crucial.**
Access to comprehensive fertility care, support services, and resources is vital for people and couples navigating infertility. Addressing financial barriers, decreasing stigma, and advocating inclusive healthcare policy are essential steps in providing equitable access to care for all.

4. **Holistic approaches to care are beneficial:**
Holistic techniques that integrate medical treatments with emotional support, counselling, nutrition, and alternative therapies can boost overall well-being and fertility outcomes. Recognizing the interdependence of physical, emotional, and psychological wellness is crucial to holistic fertility care.

5. **Advancements in Reproductive Medicine Offer Hope:**
Technological developments in assisted reproductive

technologies (ART), fertility preservation procedures, and genetic testing have transformed fertility treatment options. These developments give hope to individuals and couples battling infertility, expanding possibilities for family-building.

6. **Education and awareness are empowering.**

Fertility education, awareness campaigns, and advocacy initiatives play a significant role in decreasing stigma, enhancing knowledge, and empowering individuals to make informed decisions regarding their reproductive health. Open conversation and destigmatization lead to supportive communities and inclusive healthcare practices.

7. **Resilience and Support Foster Hope:**

Infertility can be a tough and solitary experience, but resilience, perseverance, and support from loved ones, healthcare providers, and peer communities create hope and resilience. Sharing experiences, seeking support, and accessing resources can help individuals and couples negotiate the ups and downs of infertility with courage and tenacity.

In conclusion, tackling the complex issues of infertility requires a holistic approach that incorporates medical, emotional, social, and policy dimensions. By creating awareness, advocacy, access to care, and supportive communities, we can strive towards a future where individuals and couples battling infertility are empowered, supported, and treated with dignity and compassion on their path to parenthood.